My Busy Feet

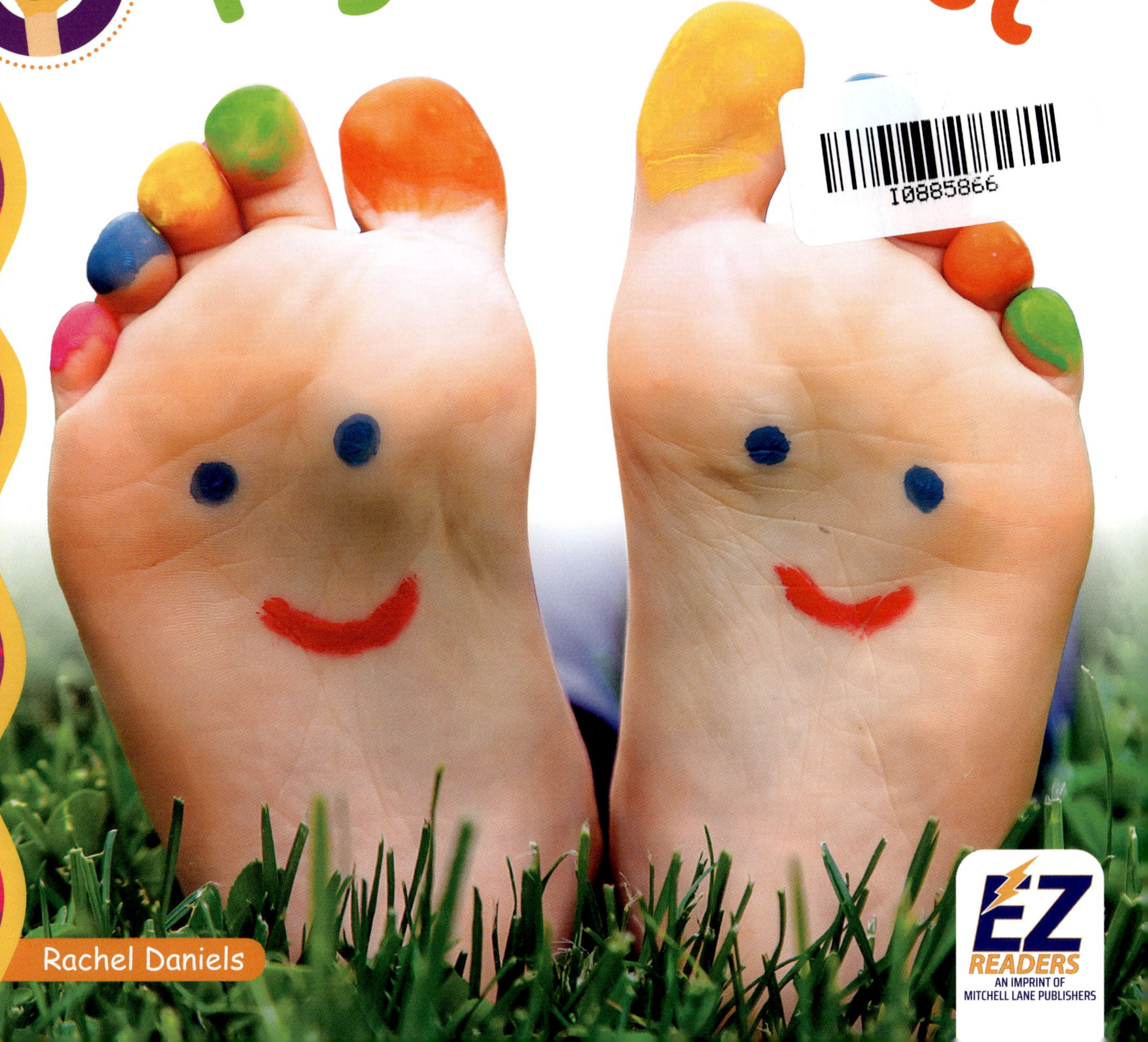

MY BODY AND ME

Rachel Daniels

EZ READERS
AN IMPRINT OF
MITCHELL LANE PUBLISHERS

CREATING YOUNG NONFICTION READERS

EZ Readers offer nonfiction for beginning readers in PreK through first grade, using simple language, clear illustrations, and engaging facts to build vocabulary and confidence.

TIPS FOR READING NONFICTION WITH BEGINNING READERS

Talk about Nonfiction

Begin by explaining that nonfiction books give us information that is true. The book will be organized around a specific topic or idea, and we may learn new facts through reading.

Look at the Parts

Most nonfiction books have helpful features. Our *EZ Readers* include color photographs and graphic aids, a table of contents, a glossary, and an index. Share the purpose of these features with your reader.

Color Photos and Graphic Aids

A lot of information can be found by "reading" photos, charts, maps, and other graphic aids found within nonfiction texts. Help your reader learn more about the different ways information can be displayed.

Table of Contents

Located at the front of the book, this list shows the big ideas within the text and the page numbers where they can be found.

Glossary

Located at the back of the book, the glossary defines key words and phrases that are related to the topic. These words and phrases can be found in the text in colored type.

Index

Located at the back of the book, an index is an alphabetical list of topics and the page numbers where they can be found.

With a little help and guidance about reading nonfiction, you can feel good about introducing a young reader to the world of *EZ Readers* nonfiction books.

EZ Readers is an imprint of:

Mitchell Lane PUBLISHERS

2001 SW 31st Avenue
Hallandale, FL 33009
mitchelllanepub.com

First Edition, 2026.

Author: Rachel Daniels
Editor: Morgan Brody

ISBN 979-8-89260-826-8 (library binding)
ISBN 979-8-90145-032-1 (paperback)
ISBN 979-8-89260-833-6 (ebook)

LC record available at https://lccn.loc.gov/2025950837

Photo credits: Shutterstock, Alex Konon, cover, 1, 2, 3, 7, 12, 16, 20; yusuf_demirci, cover, 1; Tatevosian Yana, cover, 1; Evgeny Atamanenko, 5, 22; Sergey Novikov, 6; Irina WS, 8–9; Olena Shvets, 10, 22; Roman Samborskyi, 13, 22; FamVeld, 14–15, 22; BestPhotoStudio, 17, 22; matimix, 19; SKT Studio, 21, 22; vaalaa, 22; Freepik, juicy_fish, 3, 14, 17

Table of Contents

Busy Feet Go

I have busy feet.

They run fast and hop high.

Step, step, go!

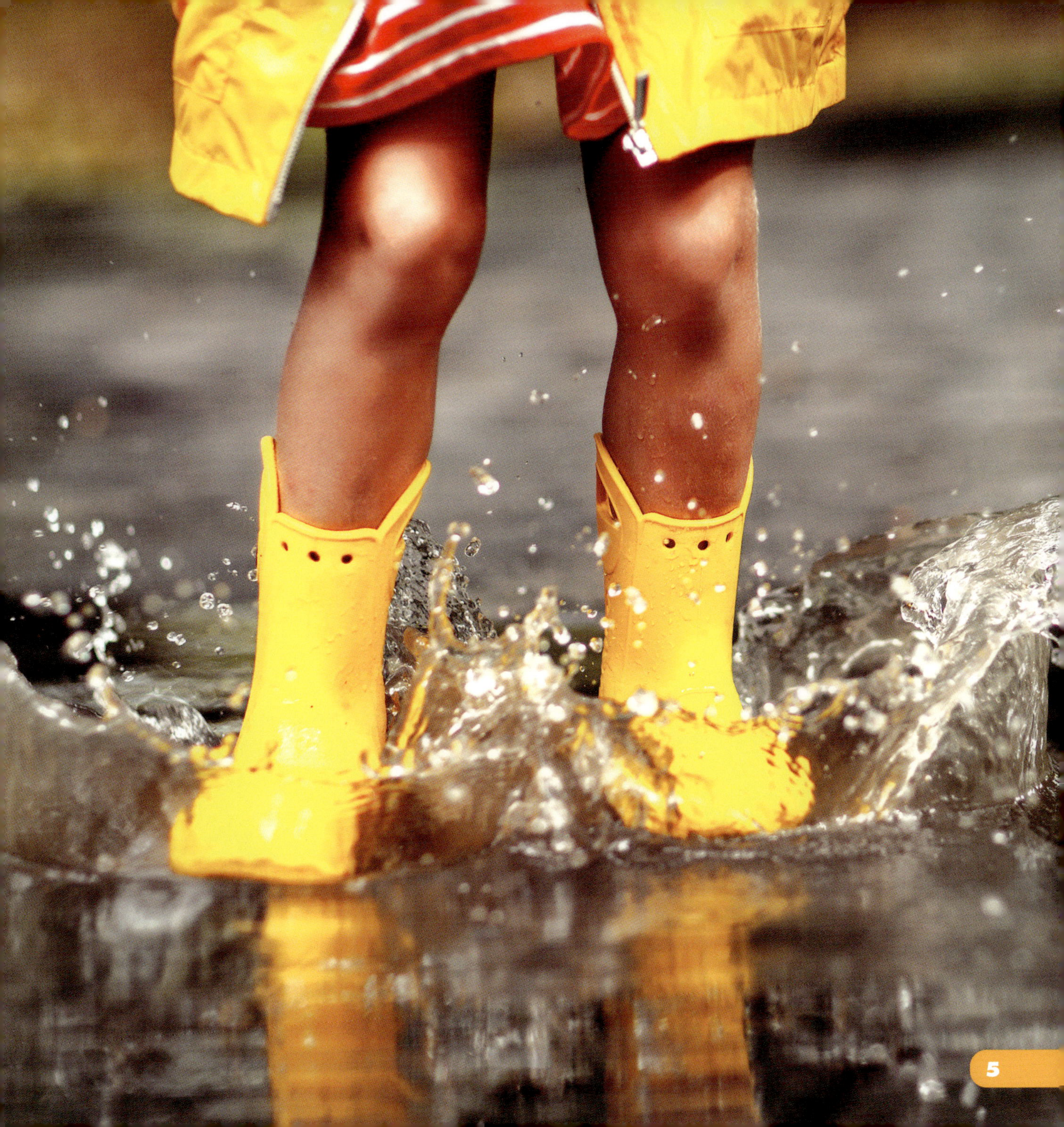

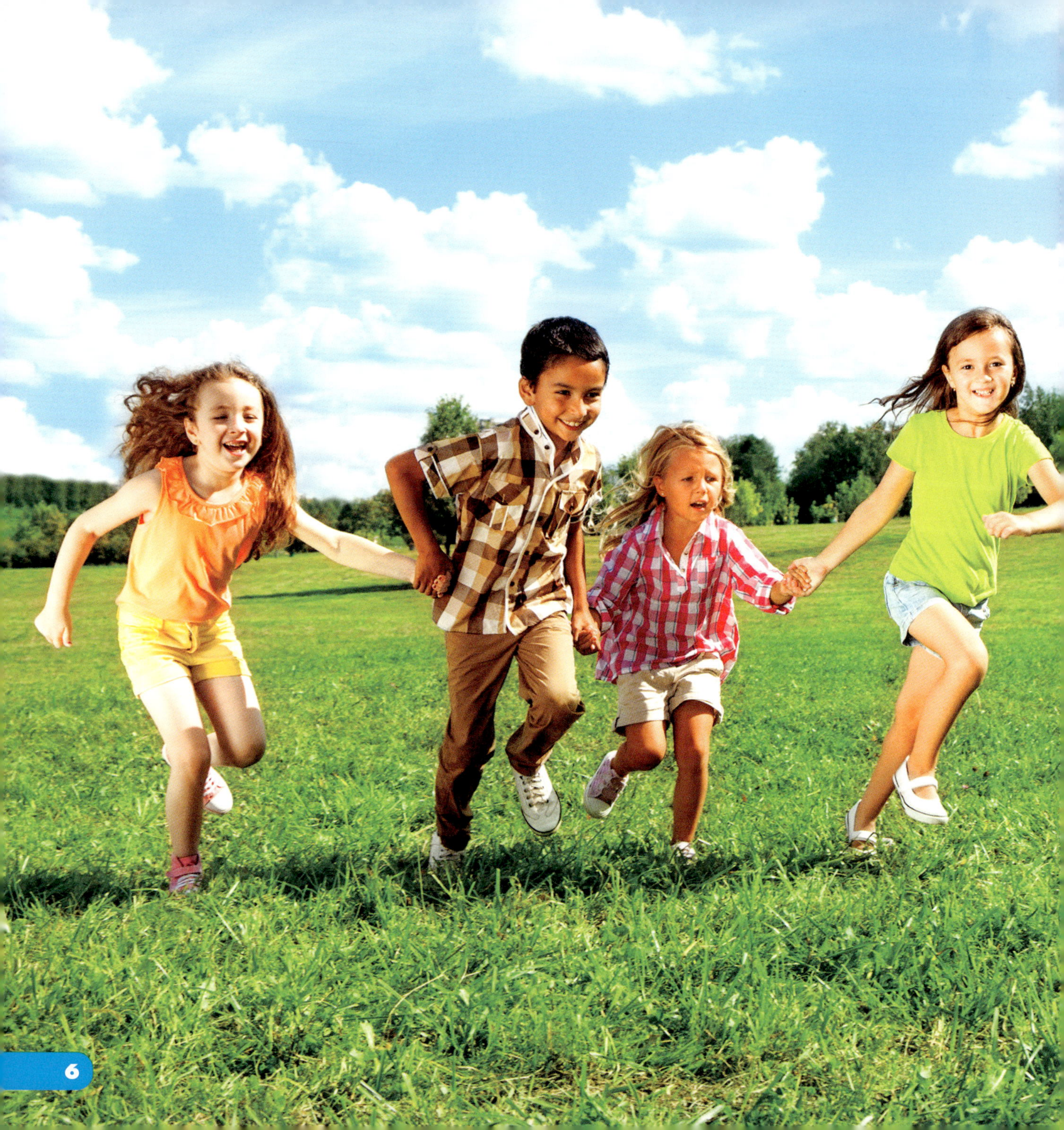

Walk and Run

I can walk slowly.

I can run very fast.

My busy feet zoom across the yard.

I hop on one foot.
I jump up high.
Boing, boing, boing!
My feet are strong.

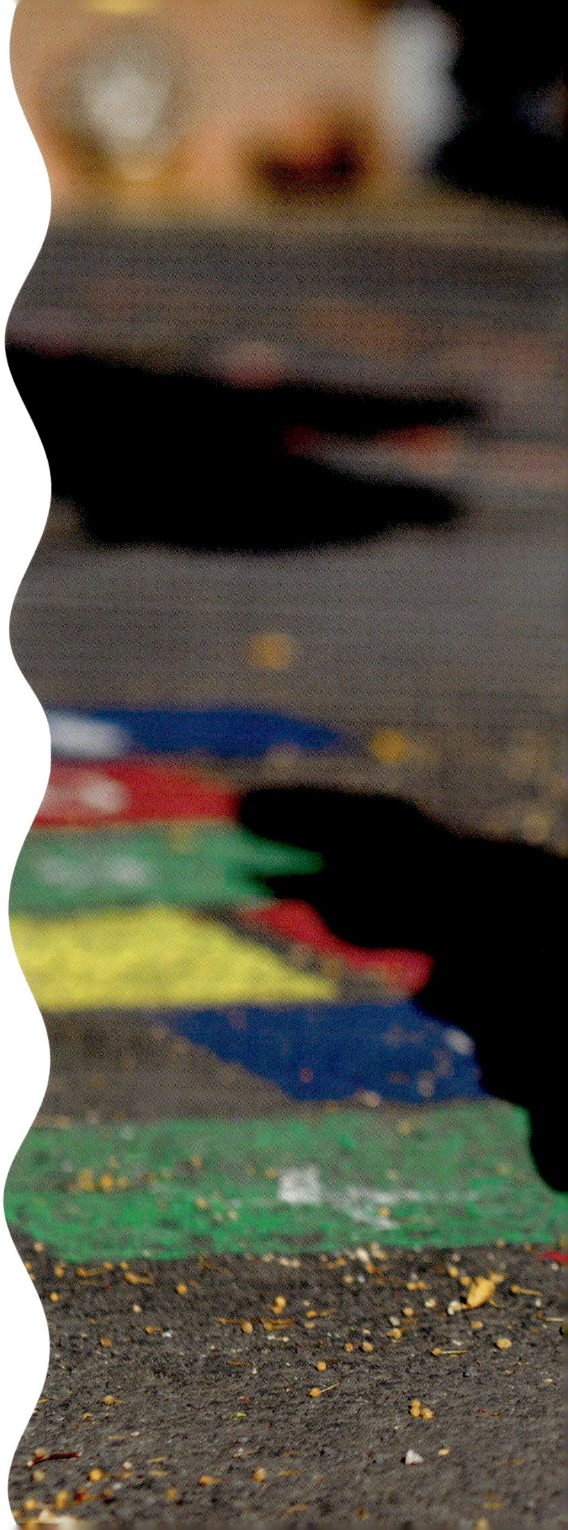

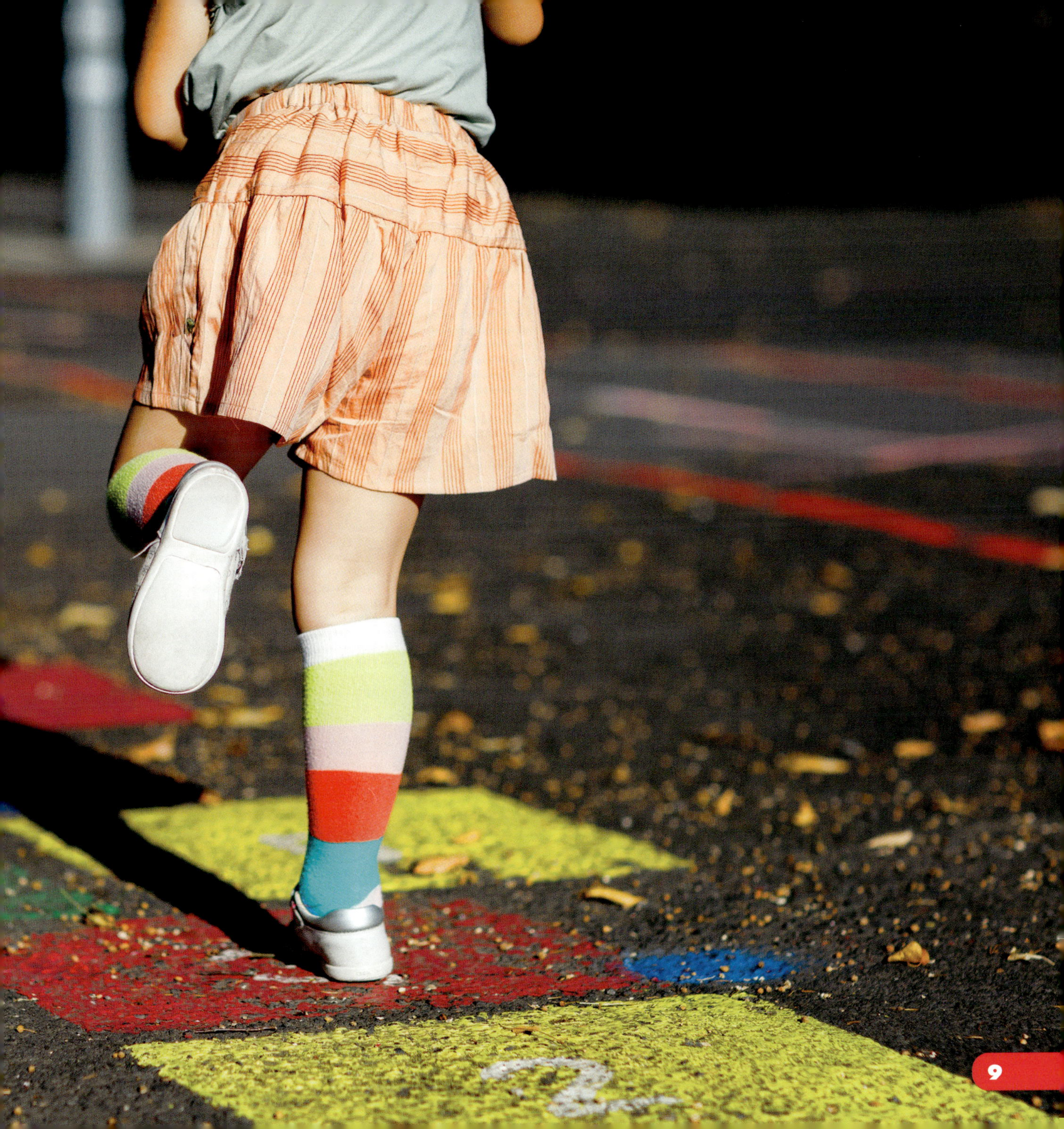
2

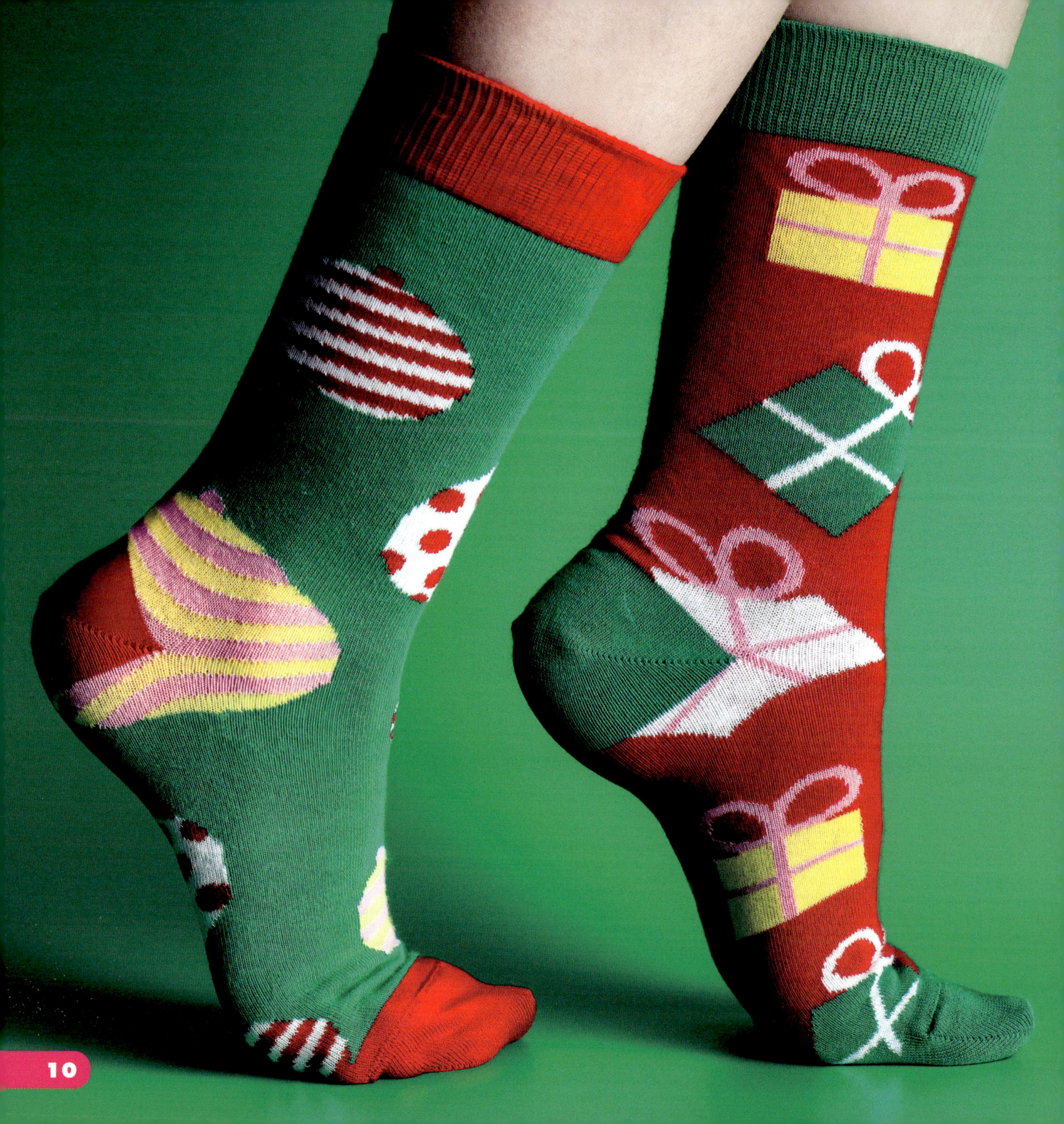

I **tiptoe** softly.

I **stomp** loudly.

Quiet feet. Loud feet.

My feet love to move!

Dance and Play

I kick a ball.

I spin and dance.

Feet help me move.

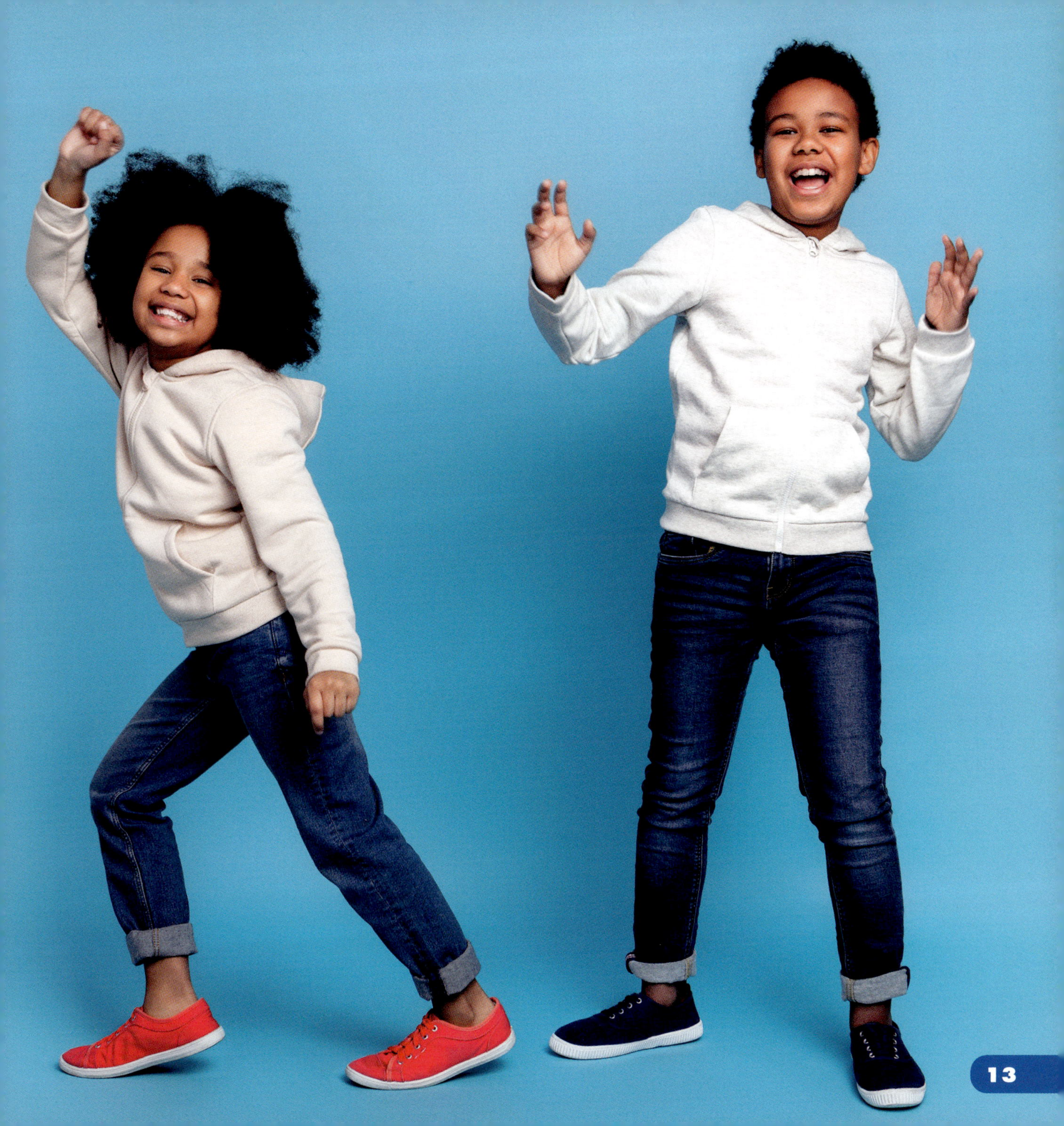

FUN FEET!

Dancers **twirl** with their busy feet.

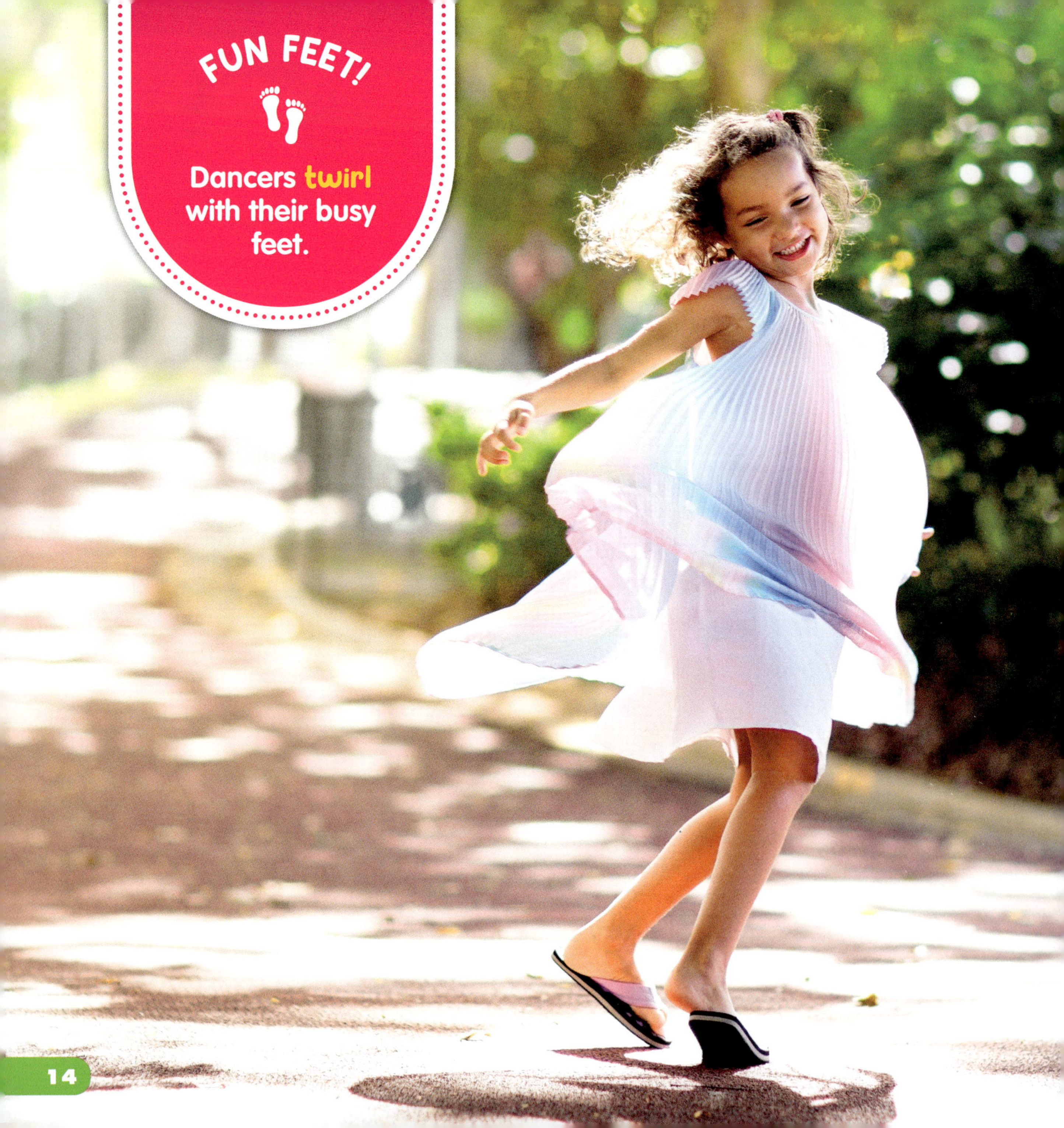

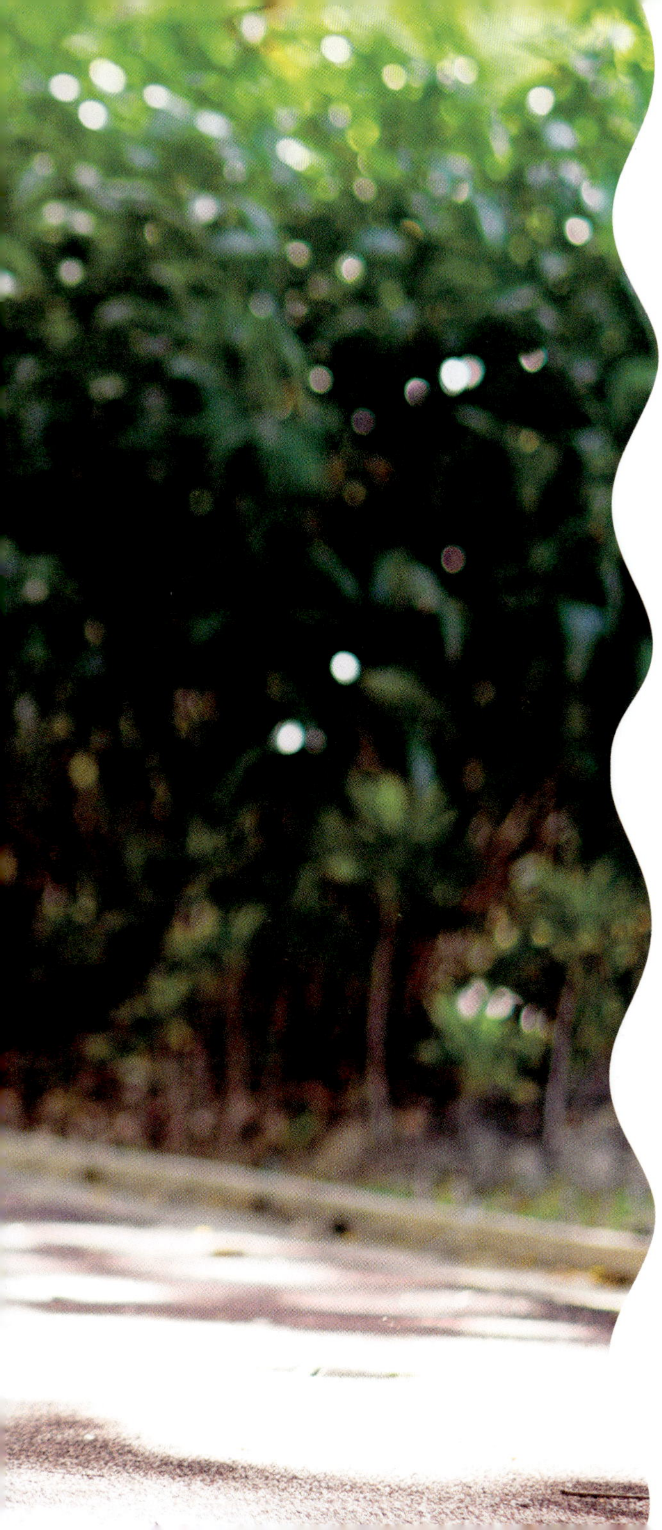

I spin in circles.

Round and round
my feet go.

Feet help me turn
safely.

Balance and Stand

I stand tall.

I **balance** on my two feet.

My feet keep me **steady**.

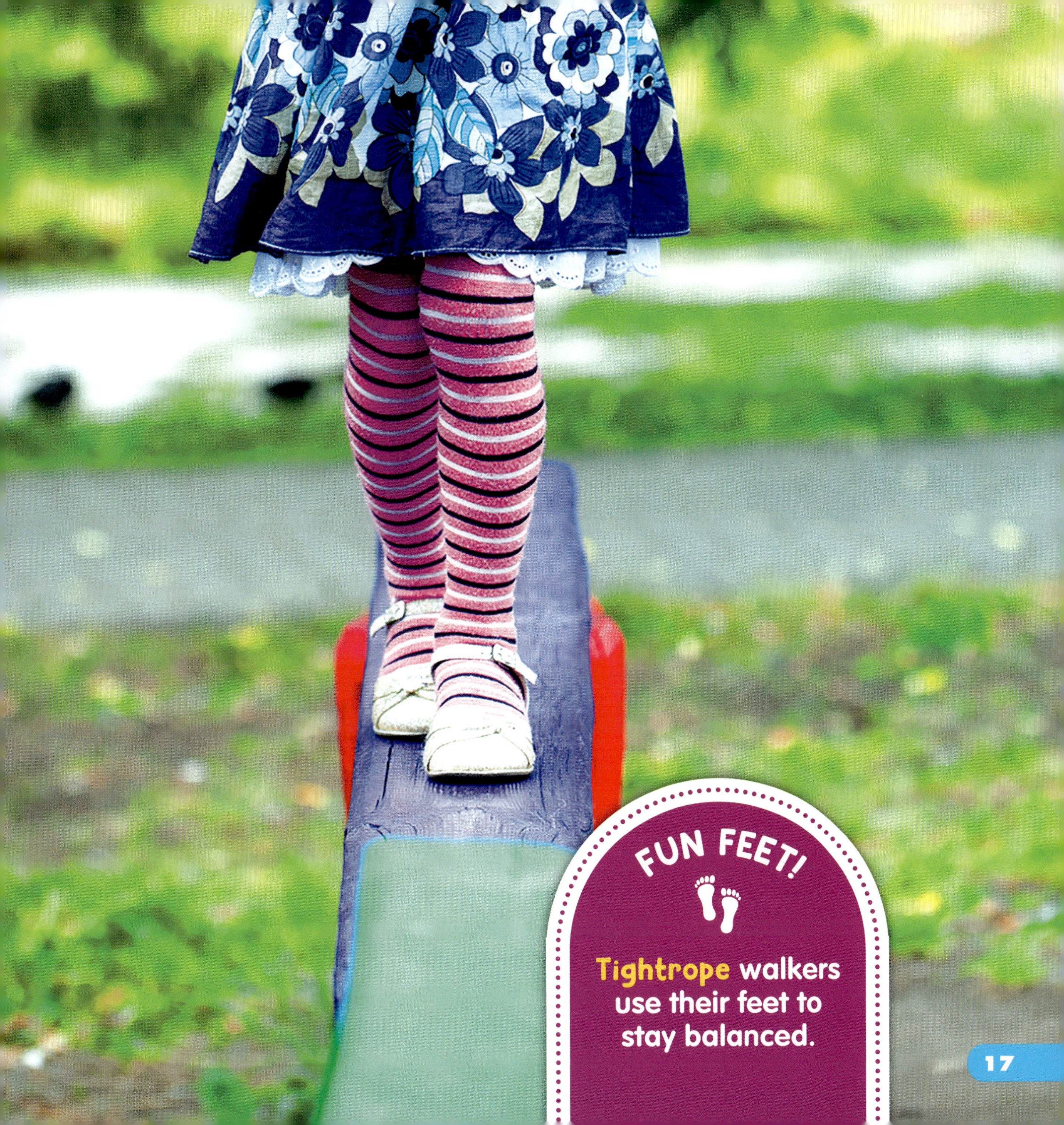

FUN FEET!

Tightrope walkers use their feet to stay balanced.

Feet run, hop, and jump.

Feet kick and stomp.

Feet help me play.

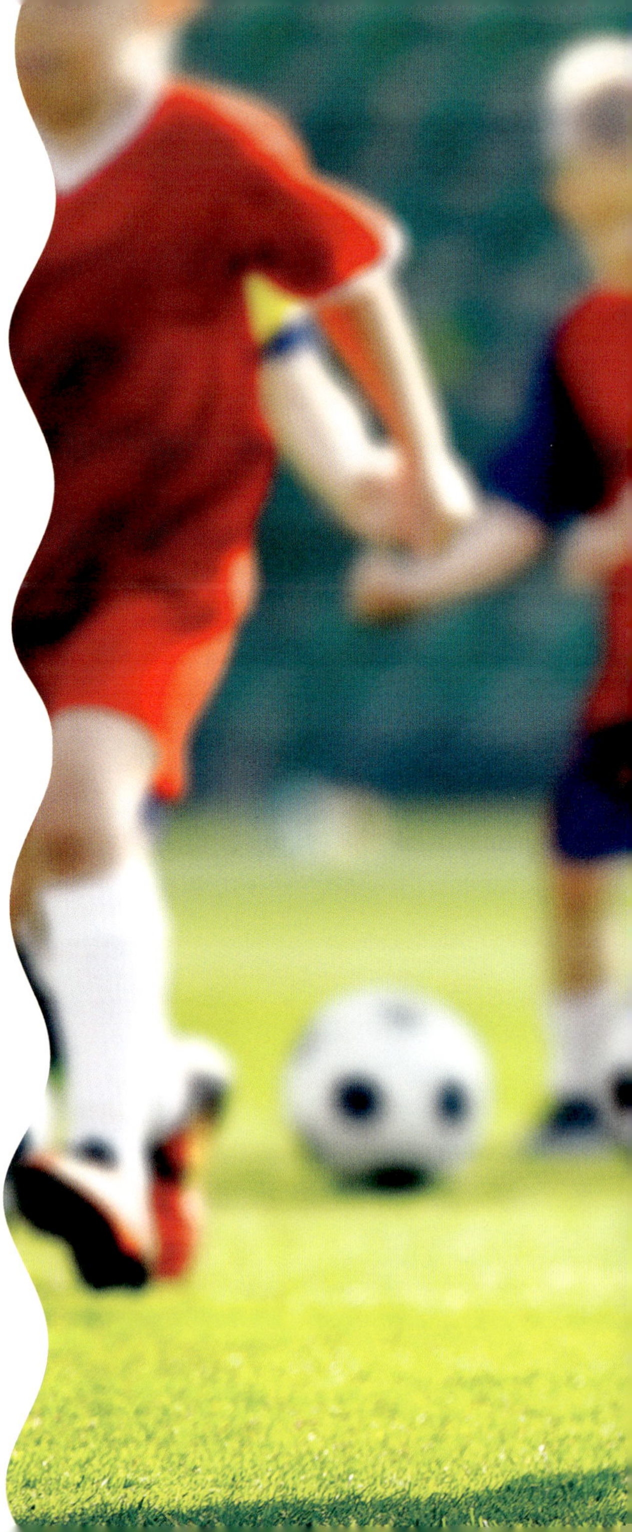

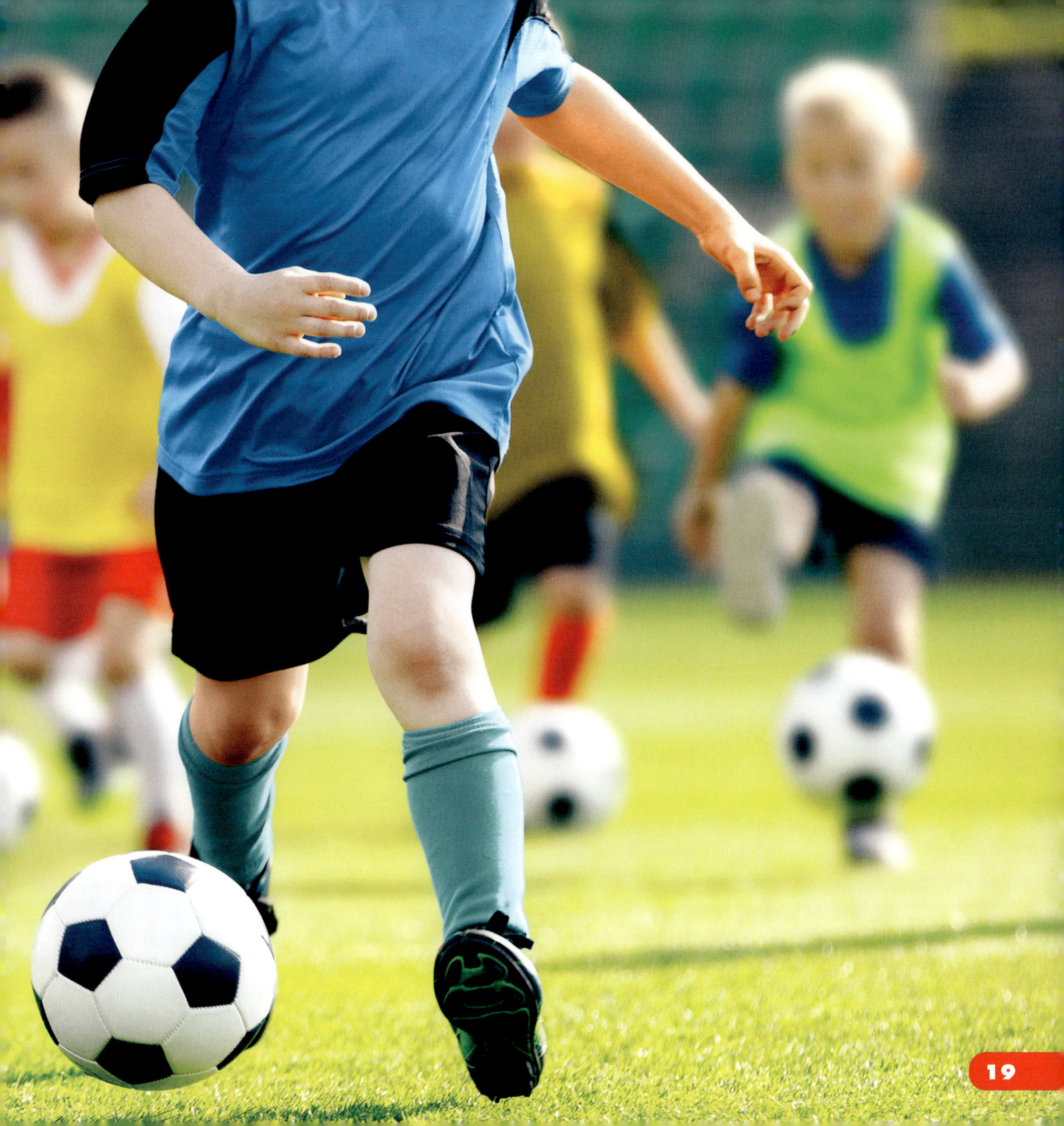

Resting Feet

At night my feet get tired.

They stop moving.

Feet rest and sleep.

Tomorrow my busy feet
will play again.

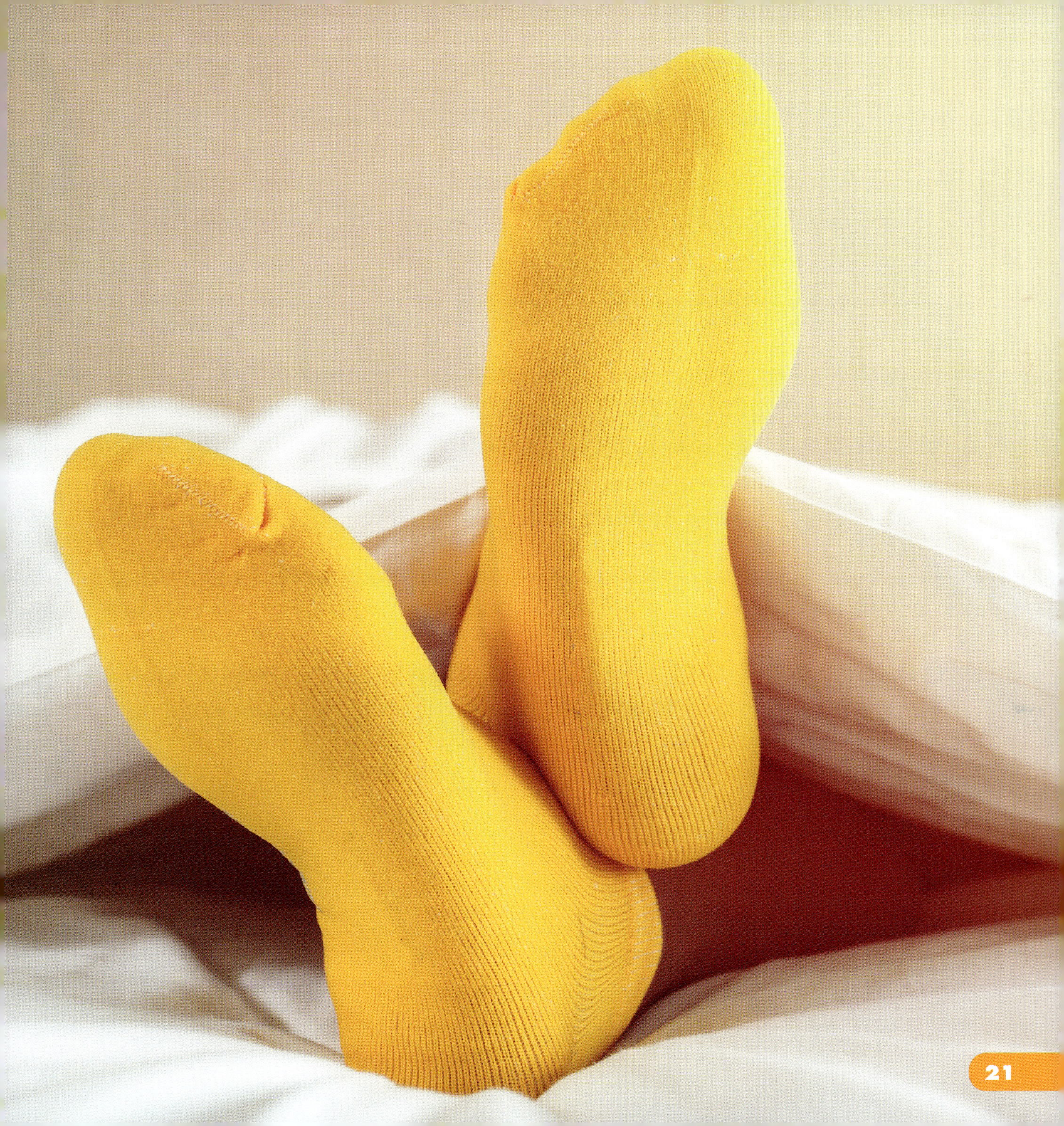

Glossary

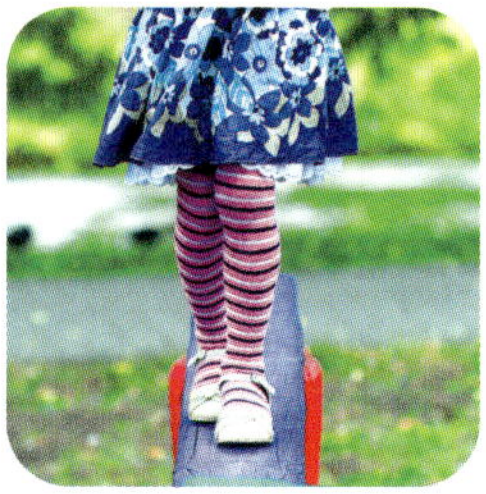

balance (BAL-anss) to stay up without falling

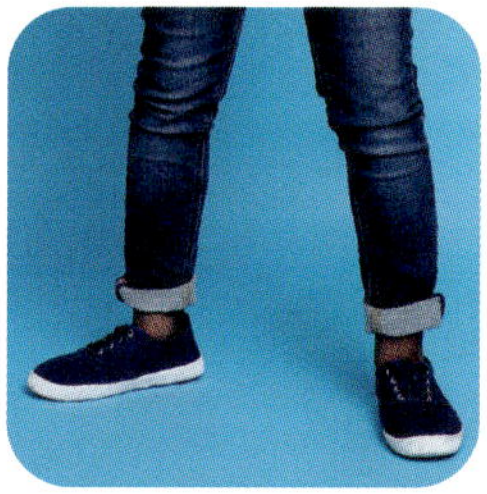

steady (STED-ee) not wobbling; staying in one place

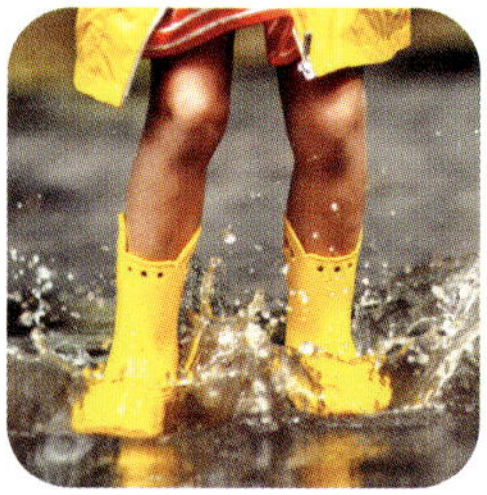

stomp (STOMP) to step down hard with your foot

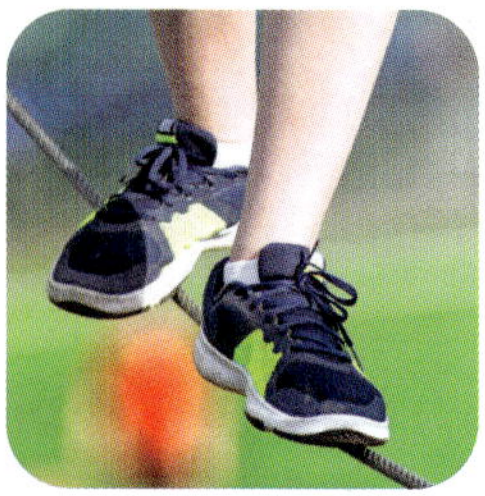

tightrope (tahyt-rohp) a rope or wire stretched high up that people walk across for a show

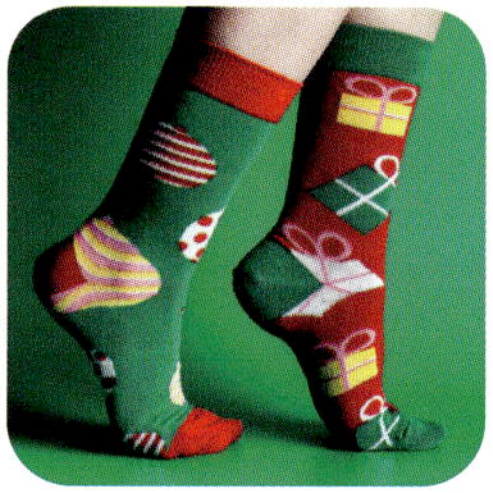

tiptoe (TIP-toe) to walk very quietly on your toes

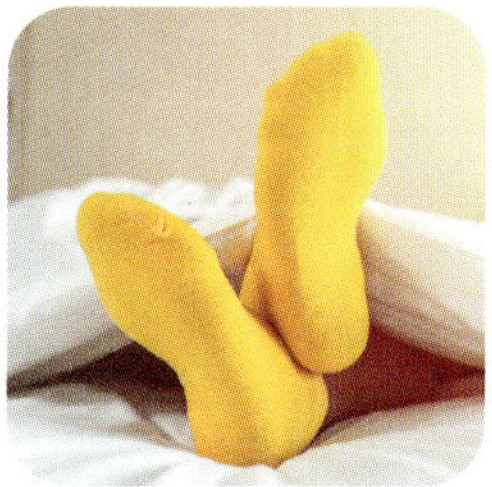

tomorrow (to-MOR-row) the day after today

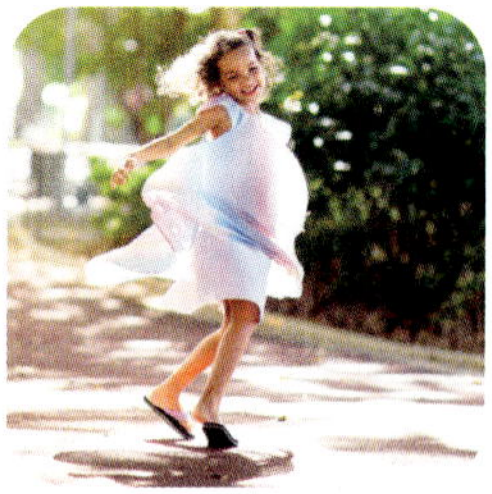

twirl (TWURL) to spin around in a circle

Quiz: My Busy Feet

1. Can feet help you balance?

A. Yes B. No

2. Do busy feet help you move all day?

A. Yes B. No

3. Can feet help you spin and twirl?

A. Yes B. No

4. Do busy feet need rest at night?

A. Yes B. No

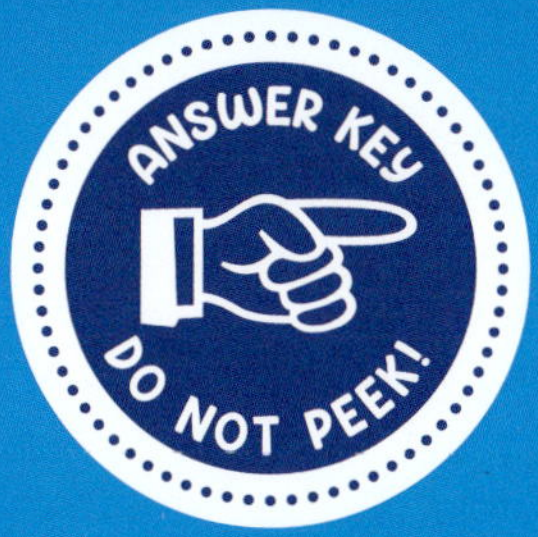

ANSWER KEY:

How many times did you answer yes?

4 Yes: Awesome! You know your busy feet really well.

3 Yes: Great! You learned lots about feet.

2 Yes: That's okay! Keep moving and learning.

1 Yes: You're just getting started. Keep going!

Further Reading

Berneger, Marcia. *Busy Feet.* Starry Forest Books, 2023.

Seuss, Dr. *The Foot Book.* Random House Children's Books, 1968.

On the Internet

KidsSoup—Hands & Feet Activities, Rhymes, and Games
https://www.kidssoup.com/activity/hands-and-feet-activities-crafts-rhymes-and-books
This site offers creative activities and movement games centered on hands and feet—great for gross motor development and body awareness.

The Inspired Treehouse—Going Barefoot: 10 Fun Activities for Kids
https://theinspiredtreehouse.com/going-barefoot-10-fun-activities-kids
A playful guide packed with barefoot movement ideas—from hopping and crawling to walking on toes or heels.

Homegrown Friends—Painting with Feet
https://homegrownfriends.com/home/painting-with-feet
A hands-on art project that invites kids to paint using their feet—engaging their sense of touch and developing gross motor skills.

Index

About the Author

Rachel Daniels is a former elementary school teacher who loves reading and discovering new things. She lives in sunny South Florida with her husband, close to her children and grandchildren. When she's not reading or writing, she enjoys playing Canasta with friends. Her goal is to make learning exciting and joyful for young readers everywhere.